ENDOMORPH DIET AND EXERCISE PLAN 2024

A 14-Day Meal Plan with Easy Exercises & Tasty Recipes to Boost Metabolism, Burn Fat & Lose Weight to Improve Your Shape & Maximize Fitness Goals.

Vince Cruise Sant

Copyright © 2023

All Rights Are Reserved

The content in this book may not be reproduced, duplicated, or transferred without the express written permission of the author or publisher. Under no circumstances will the publisher or author be held liable or legally responsible for any losses, expenditures, or damages incurred directly or indirectly as a consequence of the information included in this book.

Legal Remarks

Copyright protection applies to this publication. It is only intended for personal use. No piece of this work may be modified, distributed, sold, quoted, or paraphrased without the author's or publisher's consent.

Disclaimer Statement

Please keep in mind that the contents of this booklet are meant for educational and recreational purposes. Every effort has been made to offer accurate, up-to-date, reliable, and thorough information. There are, however, no stated or implied assurances of any kind. Readers understand that the author is providing competent counsel. The content in this book originates from several sources. Please seek the opinion of a competent professional before using any of the tactics outlined in this book. By reading this book, the reader agrees that the author will not be held accountable for any direct or indirect damages resulting from the use of the information contained therein, including, but not limited to, errors, omissions, or inaccuracies.

About The Author

Introducing Vince Cruise Sant, a seasoned nutritionist with over a decade of dedicated experience in transforming lives through the power of balanced nutrition. With an extensive background in the field, Vince has emerged as a respected figure, dedicated to guiding individuals toward achieving their health and wellness aspirations.

With a wealth of practical knowledge and a deep understanding of nutrition and metabolism, Vince's expertise extends beyond theory. Having positively impacted the lives of more than 300 individuals, he stands as a testament to the tangible results his guidance brings.

Vince's approach transcends the conventional, recognizing the individuality of each person's journey toward well-being. His methodology seamlessly blends scientific insights with real-world application, ensuring that his advice is not only attainable but also sustainable.

Recognized as a trusted advisor and advocate for balanced nutrition, Vince Cruise Sant's commitment to empowering individuals is unwavering. His reputation as a compassionate and knowledgeable guide underscores his dedication to helping others unlock their full potential.

Whether you're a newcomer to the path of wellness or seeking to refine your existing practices, Vince's expertise will inspire and educate. Prepare to embark on a transformative journey led by a visionary who firmly believes that vibrant health is an achievable reality. With Vince's guidance, your pursuit of lasting well-being is poised for exceptional success.

TABLE OF CONTENTS

INTRODUCTION **7**

Chapter 1 .... **10**

Endomorph Basics **10**

    What Exactly Is an Endomorph? 10

    Knowing Your Endomorph Body Type 10

    The Value of Tailored Approaches 13

Chapter 2 .... **17**

Setting Your Goals **17**

    Defining Your Health and Fitness Objectives 17

    Setting Realistic Endomorph Goals 21

    Monitoring Progress and Maintaining Motivation 24

Chapter 3 .... **27**

Nutrition for Endomorphs **27**

    Endomorph-Specific Nutritional Needs 27

    Designing an Endomorph Diet Plan 30

    Macronutrient Balance and Portion Control 34

    Healthy Eating Habits for Long-Term Success 37

Chapter 4 .... **42**

Meal Planning and Recipes **42**

Weekly Meal Planning for Endomorphs 42

Breakfast Recipes 52

Lunch Recipes 58

Dinner Recipes 66

Tips for Dining Out and Social Events 79

Chapter 5 84

Exercise for Endomorphs 84

Exercise's Role in Endomorph Weight Management
.... 84

Creating an Endomorph Exercise Program 87

Endomorph Cardiovascular Workouts 91

Muscle Tone Through Strength Training 94

Chapter 6 98

Workout Plans 98

12-Week Endomorph Workout Program 98

Evolution and Adaptation 103

Variation and cross-training 107

Chapter 7 111

Rest and Recovery 111

Rest is Essential for Endomorphs 111

Strategies for Effective Recovery 114

Stress and Sleep Management 118

Chapter 9 .... **122**

Additional Considerations **122**

Endomorph Supplements 122

Hormones and Weight Control 124

Conclusion **129**

INTRODUCTION

Hello and welcome to "ENDOMORPH DIET AND EXERCISE PLAN 2024." This book will help you understand, embrace, and optimize the endomorph body type's unique journey to better health, fitness, and general well-being.

In a world where one-size-fits-all solutions rule the health and fitness sector, it's critical to acknowledge that each person is delightfully unique. Understanding the variances in our bodies' shapes, sizes, and metabolic profiles is the first step in achieving long-term, sustainable health and fitness objectives.

The endomorph body type, which is distinguished by a propensity to retain fat and a naturally curvier shape, frequently encounters specific hurdles on the route to optimal health. These problems, however, are not insurmountable; rather, they represent chances for development, change, and empowerment. This book is your unique road map to reaching your health and fitness objectives, tailored to your endomorph body type.

You'll discover a thorough, up-to-date, and science-backed approach to diet and fitness on these pages. We shall delve into the complexities of the endomorph body type, from genetic predispositions to metabolic traits. You will learn to love your body, establish attainable objectives, and create a personalized strategy that works for you rather than against you.

Our purpose is simple: to offer you the information, skills, and techniques you need to reach your maximum endomorph potential. Whether you want to lose weight, gain muscle, enhance energy, or simply live a healthy lifestyle, this book has you covered.

You'll learn the secrets of endomorph-specific nutrition, such as how to develop a sustainable and fun eating plan that supports your goals. We'll go through efficient training regimens specific to your body type, which will help you burn fat, develop muscle, and increase your metabolism.

But this book is about more than simply diets and workouts. We'll also discuss the significance of relaxation, rehabilitation, and stress management—all of which are essential components of a well-balanced and long-term health and fitness plan. You'll learn how to deal with failures, conquer plateaus, and stay inspired along the way.

Furthermore, we will share real-life endomorph success stories to demonstrate how, with the correct education, determination, and support, you can make extraordinary transformations and become the healthiest and happiest version of yourself.

As we begin on this adventure together, remember that your endomorph body type is not a disadvantage; it is your distinct advantage. You may accomplish exceptional results and experience a level of health and energy that you may have believed was out of reach by utilizing your body's intrinsic qualities and adjusting your approach.

So, if you're ready to accept your endomorph physique and embark on a journey to improved health, let's get started. The "ENDOMORPH DIET AND EXERCISE PLAN 2024" is your all-encompassing guide, your dependable friend, and your key to a healthier, more vibrant self. Your journey has begun.

CHAPTER 1

ENDOMORPH BASICS

What Exactly Is an Endomorph?

Endomorphs are one of the three basic somatotypes, or body types, used to define and describe human physique variances. In the 1940s, American psychologist William H. Sheldon established the notion of somatotypes as a mechanism to categorize people based on their physical traits and body composition.

Knowing Your Endomorph Body Type

There is a wonderful range of body types in the interesting realm of human biology, each with its own set of qualities, capabilities, and problems. One such body type is the endomorph, which is differentiated from its ectomorphic and mesomorphic cousins by several fundamental characteristics. Understanding the endomorph body type is the first step toward reaching optimal health and fitness since it offers a framework for tailoring solutions.

Endomorph Characteristics:

Endomorphs have a genetic inclination to retain body fat more quickly than other body types. Endomorphs are more likely to develop fat in places such as the belly, hips, and thighs when presented with a calorie surplus.

Endomorphs have a curvier and softer look, with a rounder face and broader torso. They may be shorter in stature and have a more noticeable pear-shaped or apple-shaped profile.

Slower Metabolism: The pace at which the body consumes calories for energy is referred to as metabolism. Endomorphs have a slower metabolic rate than ectomorphs (those with a slimmer physique). This implies they may need to be more mindful of calorie consumption and more committed to exercise to maintain or reduce weight.

Endomorphs may be more prone to gaining body fat, but they also can acquire large muscle mass. They may develop a powerful, well-defined body with the correct training plan.

Endomorphs frequently struggle with the difficulty of acquiring weight more easily than other body types. This may be both a benefit and a curse since it means they might experience quick success in muscle building with the appropriate technique, but they must be careful with nutrition and activity to avoid undesirable fat gain.

Endomorph Body Type Acceptance:

It is critical to underline that being an endomorph is not a disadvantage, but rather a distinct feature with its own set of benefits. You may adjust your health and fitness plans to work with your genetic predispositions after you understand your body type. Here are some crucial items to remember:

Endomorphs should pay special attention to their food choices because they tended to retain fat. A well-balanced, nutrient-dense diet with calorie restriction can aid in weight management.

Strength Training Is Essential: Endomorphs excel in strength training and muscle growth. Incorporating resistance training into your workout program will help you increase your metabolism and enhance your body composition.

Cardiovascular activity: In addition to strength training, cardiovascular activity is essential for general health and calorie expenditure. It is critical to strike a balance between the two forms of exercise.

Patience and persistence: Endomorphs may take longer to achieve fitness and health objectives, but persistence and patience are essential. Small, long-term alterations can lead to substantial shifts.

Seek Professional Help: Working with a fitness trainer, nutritionist, or healthcare professional that knows the specific needs of endomorphs may be extremely valuable in developing a customized strategy.

The Value of Tailored Approaches

One size does not fit all when it comes to health and fitness. Tailored techniques, also known as personalized or tailored approaches, are critical for attaining the best outcomes, motivating employees, and guaranteeing long-term success. Rather than depending on generic, one-size-fits-all solutions, these techniques take into consideration an individual's unique features, requirements, objectives, and limits. Here are some of the reasons why personalized methods are so important:

Increasing Effectiveness: Everyone has a unique body type, genetics, metabolism, fitness level, and health condition. What works well for one individual may not work as well for another. A personalized strategy takes these individual aspects into account to develop a plan that enhances efficacy.

Obtaining Long-Term outcomes: Generic exercise and diet routines frequently produce short-term success but fail to produce long-term outcomes. A personalized approach considers an individual's preferences, lifestyle, and limits, increasing the likelihood that the person will remain with the plan in the long run.

Preventing Injuries and Health hazards: Forcing people to participate in activities or diets that are not appropriate for their physical capacities can result in injuries and health hazards. To guarantee safety, tailored procedures take into account a person's fitness level, current health issues, and other physical restrictions.

Individuals are more likely to stay motivated when a strategy is tailored because they see outcomes that are relevant to their unique goals. This increases compliance and increases the chance of obtaining and sustaining targeted goals.

Changing Needs: Life circumstances, health problems, and fitness objectives can all change over time. A personalized strategy is adaptable and may be altered as needed to meet these changes, preserving its relevance and effectiveness.

Taking into Account Psychological aspects: Tailored techniques can also take into account psychological aspects such as a person's thinking, preferences, and emotional relationship with food and exercise. These elements are critical to long-term success yet are frequently disregarded in general strategies.

Time and Resource Optimization: Not everyone has the same amount of time or access to the same resources. A personalized strategy is more realistic and achievable since it takes into consideration an individual's available time, finances, and access to equipment or facilities.

Improving Overall Well-Being: Health and fitness should be about more than just looks or performance. A personalized approach can take into account a person's complete well-being, such as mental health, stress levels, and quality of life, resulting in a more holistic and enjoyable journey.

Individual Empowerment: Individuals feel more empowered and aware of their health and fitness by participating in the formulation of a customized plan. This sense of empowerment promotes a sense of ownership and responsibility for one's well-being.

Recognizing and valuing the diversity of individuals and their distinct requirements is not only ethical but also a cornerstone of good healthcare and fitness practices.

CHAPTER 2

SETTING YOUR GOALS

Defining Your Health and Fitness Objectives

Defining your health and fitness goals is an important first step toward a better and more active lifestyle. Clear goals give direction, motivation, and a structure for organizing your exercise and health program. Here's a detailed guide to defining your health and fitness goals:

1. Self-Evaluation:

existing Health Status: Begin by examining your existing state of health and fitness. Consider your weight, body composition, blood pressure, cholesterol levels, and other medical concerns you may have. This baseline evaluation will assist you in determining your present position.

Strength, flexibility, endurance, and balance are examples of physical characteristics to consider. Make a list of any restrictions or places where you would wish to improve.

Reflect on your everyday habits, such as nutrition, exercise, sleep, and stress management. Determine where you can make improvements.

2. Establish Specific Objectives: Make your objectives explicit and well-defined. Instead of a general objective like "lose weight," describe how much weight you want to lose and when you want to lose it.

Goals should be quantifiable so that you can measure your progress. Use measures such as weight loss, inches gained, or workout frequency.

Achievable: Make sure your objectives are both practical and reachable. Set goals that are within your reach to set yourself up for success.

Relevant: Your objectives should be related to your life and ideals. They should be in line with your priorities.

Time-Bound: Assign a completion date to your goals. This creates a sense of urgency and aids in your accountability. For example, set a goal of reaching a specific level of fitness in three months.

3. Examine Various Aspects of Health and Fitness: Physical Fitness: Establish physical fitness goals, such as increasing cardiovascular endurance, strength, flexibility, or balance.

Set dietary goals, such as consuming a particular number of servings of fruits and vegetables per day, lowering your sugar intake, or preparing more meals at home.

Weight Management: If you are concerned about your weight, create weight-related objectives such as decreasing a specific amount of pounds or maintaining a healthy weight range.

Mental and Emotional Health: Don't overlook your mental and emotional well-being. Consider stress reduction, improved sleep, or mindfulness activities as goals.

4. Prioritize Your Objectives: Sort your goals according to their significance. This allows you to focus on the most important goals while avoiding overload.

5. Develop an Action Plan: Divide your ambitions into smaller, more manageable tasks. For example, if you want to run a marathon, you may start with a couch-to-5k program, progressively increase your mileage, and participate in lesser events as milestones.

Consider the resources, time, and assistance required to attain each objective.

6. Monitor and Adjust: Track your progress regularly with a diary, fitness app, or spreadsheet. Keep track of your triumphs and failures.

Be willing to make changes. If you discover that a goal is either too difficult or not tough enough, alter it as required.

7. Maintain Accountability: Share your objectives with a friend, family member, or coach who can help you stay on track.

For added support and encouragement, consider joining a workout club, class, or online community.

8. Commemorate Milestones: Along the journey, celebrate your accomplishments. When you hit milestones, recognize and congratulate yourself, but avoid using food as a reward.

9. Reassess and Set New Goals: As you achieve your first goals, evaluate your progress and establish new targets regularly. This keeps you motivated and guarantees that you continue to grow and progress.

Setting Realistic Endomorph Goals

Setting realistic goals is vital for people of all body types, especially endomorphs. Setting health and fitness goals as an endomorph requires taking into account your body's specific qualities and limitations. Here are some pointers to help you create realistic objectives as an endomorph:

1. Accept Realistic Expectations: Recognize that your progress may be slower than that of other body types. Endomorphs may require a longer time to achieve apparent results due to their proclivity to accumulate fat.

2. Concentrate on Body Composition: Rather than focusing exclusively on weight loss, look for changes in body composition. This includes increasing lean muscle mass and lowering body fat, which can result in a more youthful appearance.

3. Establish both short-term and long-term objectives: Divide your ultimate aim into smaller, more manageable benchmarks. This gives you a sense of success and keeps you motivated along the road.

4. Set SMART objectives: Specific: Clearly explain your objectives.

Measurable measures, such as body fat percentage or inches loss, should be used.

Achievable: Set goals that are within your reach, taking into account your body type and starting position.

Make sure your objectives are relevant to your health and fitness priorities.

Time-Bound: Set a realistic timetable for completing each objective.

5. Concentrate on Small-Scale Victories: Celebrate milestones that go beyond the scale, such as increased stamina, strength, flexibility, and energy levels.

6. Make nutrition a priority: Set nutritional objectives that stress balanced eating, portion management, and eating healthier foods.

7. Weight Loss in Small Steps: If you want to lose weight, strive for a slow and sustained rate of 0.5 to 1 pound each week. Rapid weight reduction might result in muscle loss and a decrease in metabolism.

8. Include Strength Training: Set goals for strength training and muscular growth. Endomorphs can successfully grow muscle, which can raise metabolism and improve body composition.

9. Incorporate Cardiovascular Exercise: Cardiovascular exercise is critical for heart health and calorie expenditure. Set objectives for regular cardiovascular activities to help with weight loss.

10. Track Progress: Take measurements, photographs, and keep a fitness journal to document your progress. This allows you to notice beneficial improvements even if they aren't immediately visible.

11. Be Consistent and Patient: Recognize that development takes time. Maintain your commitment to your goals and have faith in the process.

12. Seek Professional Help: Consult with a fitness trainer or dietitian who has worked with endomorphs before. They can assist you in developing a customized plan and give professional advice.

Monitoring Progress and Maintaining Motivation

Regardless of your body type, effective progress monitoring and motivation are critical components of reaching your health and fitness goals. As an endomorph, it is very crucial to regularly assess your progress to stay on track and enthused. Here are some techniques to help you successfully measure your progress and maintain your motivation:

1. Establish clear and specific goals:

Setting specific and well-defined goals gives you a clear feeling of purpose. Make sure your objectives are precise, measurable, attainable, relevant, and time-bound (SMART).

2. Keep a Fitness Journal:

Maintain a notebook in which you record your exercises, nutritional choices, and general health. This notebook can assist you in tracking your progress and identifying trends in your health and fitness journey.

3. Take Measurements regularly:

Measure crucial variables such as your weight, body fat percentage, waist circumference, and muscle mass to track physical changes. Consistency in measuring conditions (for example, same time of day, same outfit) guarantees reliable results.

4. Keep track of non-scale accomplishments:

Celebrate achievements that go beyond the numbers on the scale, such as increased endurance, strength, flexibility, and energy levels. These successes can operate as tremendous motivators.

5. Make Use of Technology:

Track your progress, calculate calories, and record your exercises using fitness apps, wearable gadgets, and internet resources. Many of these applications also provide visually shown representations of your progress, which may be quite encouraging.

6. Photograph Progress:

Take photographs of yourself in consistent lighting and positions regularly to visibly track your body's alterations over time. Seeing bodily gains may be a powerful incentive.

7. Create a Reward System:

Make a system in which you reward yourself for hitting certain goals. These prizes should be in line with your fitness goals (e.g., avoid using unhealthy foods as rewards) and might include items such as new training gear, a spa day, or a fun excursion.

8. Discuss Your Goals:

Discuss your fitness and health objectives with a friend, family member, or exercise partner. Accountability can be a powerful motivator, and having someone with whom you can discuss your successes and struggles can help you stay engaged.

9. Participate in a Helpful Community:

Participate in fitness forums, social media groups, or local fitness clubs to meet people with similar interests. Participating in a community may boost motivation by building friendships and providing support.

CHAPTER 3

NUTRITION FOR ENDOMORPHS

Endomorph-Specific Nutritional Needs

Endomorphs have special dietary demands that can help them reach and maintain a healthy body composition because of their genetic inclination to accumulate body fat more quickly. Here are some dietary requirements and explanations for endomorphs:

1. Macronutrients in Balance:

Endomorphs benefit from a well-balanced macronutrient ratio. This usually entails eating a diet with a reasonable quantity of carbs, proteins, and healthy fats. A well-balanced macronutrient intake can aid in blood sugar regulation and energy balance.

2. Carbohydrates Under Control:

Endomorphs should pay special attention to their carbohydrate intake. Choose complex carbs over refined sugars and processed grains, such as whole grains, vegetables, and legumes. This aids in the stabilization of blood sugar levels and the prevention of excessive fat buildup.

3. Portion Management:

Endomorphs should watch their portion sizes since they are more prone to accumulating extra calories as fat. Eating smaller, more balanced meals throughout the day can assist in controlling calorie intake and metabolism.

4. Consistent Eating Routine:

A regular meal schedule can help balance blood sugar levels and minimize overeating, which is especially important for endomorphs, who are prone to weight gain.

5. Foods High in Fiber:

Fiber-rich foods, such as fruits, vegetables, and whole grains, are full and can aid with hunger control. They help promote intestinal health, which is essential for general health.

6. Lean Proteins:

Protein is necessary for muscle maintenance and can also aid with appetite management. Choose lean protein sources such as poultry, fish, tofu, and lentils while limiting higher-fat protein alternatives.

7. Good Fats: Avocados, almonds, seeds, and olive oil are all good sources of healthful fats. Healthy fats are satiating and supplying necessary nutrients while also aiding with calorie control.

8. Reduced Sugar Consumption:

Reduce your intake of added sugars, which can cause blood sugar spikes and crashes and perhaps increase fat accumulation. Be wary of sugary drinks and processed meals.

9. Hydration

Hydration is essential for metabolism and general health. Water consumption throughout the day can aid in appetite management and assist the body's natural fat-burning activities.

10. Consistent Meals and Snacks:

Avoid missing meals and try to incorporate nutritious snacks in between. This helps to keep blood sugar levels steady, minimizes the probability of overeating, and promotes consistent energy levels.

11. Reduced Processed Foods: Processed foods are frequently high in hidden sugars, harmful fats, and calories. Reducing your consumption of processed and quick meals can help you regulate your calorie intake.

12. Personalized Approach:

It's crucial to keep in mind that, while these broad guidelines are useful, individual dietary demands might differ greatly. Some endomorphs may benefit from slightly varied macronutrient ratios or have specialized dietary preferences. A certified dietitian or nutritionist who specializes in personalized meal planning can be quite useful.

13. Patience and consistency:

It takes effort and consistency to achieve and maintain healthy body composition. Maintain your patience and commitment to your dietary plan, and be ready to make changes as needed depending on your success.

Designing an Endomorph Diet Plan

Creating a diet plan for your endomorph body type entails selecting particular food choices that benefit your metabolism, body composition objectives, and general health. Here's a step-by-step method for developing an endomorph food plan:

1. **Determine Your Caloric Requirements:** Calculate your daily calorie needs depending on your age, gender, amount of exercise, and goals (for example, weight reduction or muscle building). Many internet calculators can assist you in estimating this.

2. **Macronutrient Balance:** Aim for a well-balanced macronutrient consumption. A decent starting point is a ratio of roughly 40% carbs, 30% protein, and 30% healthy fats. These ratios should be adjusted based on your tastes and how your body reacts.

3. **Opt for Complex Carbohydrates:** Choose complex carbs such as whole grains (brown rice, quinoa, whole wheat), veggies, and legumes above simple carbohydrates. These give prolonged energy and aid in the stabilization of blood sugar levels, hence minimizing fat formation.

4. **Incorporate Lean Proteins:** Prioritize chicken, fish, lean cuts of beef or pig, tofu, tempeh, and legumes as lean protein sources. Protein aids with muscle maintenance and hunger management.

5. Good Fats: Include healthy fats from avocados, nuts, seeds, olive oil, and fatty fish (salmon, mackerel) in your diet. These fats supply necessary nutrients while also increasing satiety.

6. Portion Management: Be aware of portion sizes, especially when eating high-calorie items. If necessary, use measuring cups and a food scale until you have a strong understanding of proper portion sizes.

7. Consume Fiber-Rich Foods: Eat fiber-rich foods such as fruits, vegetables, and whole grains. Fiber increases satiety, assists digestion, and improves general health.

8. Control Your Sugar Intake: Reduce your intake of added sugars and processed carbs. This reduces fat accumulation by preventing blood sugar spikes and crashes.

9. Consistent Meal Scheduling: Maintain a consistent eating routine that includes three major meals and healthy snacks in between. This aids in the regulation of hunger and the maintenance of steady blood sugar levels.

10. Hydration: Drink lots of water throughout the day to stay hydrated. Thirst might be confused with hunger at times.

11. Opt for Nutrient-Dense Foods: Prioritize nutrient-dense meals that are high in vitamins and minerals yet low in calories. Leafy greens, colorful veggies, and lean meats are some examples.

12. Meal Preparation: choose meals ahead of time so that healthy selections are easily available, limiting the temptation to choose less nutritious choices when hungry.

13. Track Your Progress: Keep a food journal to document your daily consumption and see how your body reacts to various meals and meal times.

14. Seek Professional Help: Consult with an endomorph nutrition specialist, such as a certified dietitian or nutritionist. They may offer tailored advice and assist you in fine-tuning your nutrition plan to match your requirements.

15. Be Patient and Flexible: Recognize that obtaining and maintaining a healthy body composition is a slow and steady process. Be kind to yourself, and don't be afraid to change your eating plan based on your results and how your body reacts.

Macronutrient Balance and Portion Control

Portion management and macronutrient balance are critical components of a healthy diet, and they are especially crucial for those who want to lose weight, change their body composition, or meet specific nutritional objectives. Let's take a deeper look at each of these ideas:

1. Portion Management:

Portion control is the management of the amount of food consumed in a single serving or meal. It's a beneficial habit since it allows you to:

Control Caloric Intake: Portion control can help to prevent overeating and excessive calorie consumption, which is important for weight management.

Smaller amounts encourage mindful eating, in which you taste your meal and pay attention to hunger and fullness cues.

Prevent Food Waste: Proper portion control eliminates food waste by ensuring that just what you need is prepared and consumed.

Here are some helpful hints for portion control:

To naturally minimize portion sizes, use smaller dishes and bowls.

Keep an eye out for serving-size information on food labels.

To acquire a feel of acceptable servings, measure or weigh your meal beforehand.

Keep an eye out for portion distortion in restaurants, where servings are sometimes bigger than necessary.

2. Macronutrient Equilibrium:

Balancing macronutrients entails eating the proper quantities of carbs, proteins, and lipids. Each macronutrient has a distinct role to perform in your overall health and nutrition:

Carbohydrates are the body's principal energy source. Concentrate on complex carbs such as whole grains, fruits, and vegetables for fiber, vitamins, and minerals.

Proteins are required for tissue healing, muscle maintenance, and a variety of biological processes. Choose lean protein sources such as chicken, fish, beans, tofu, and low-fat dairy.

Fats: Healthy fats promote general health, including brain function and nutrient absorption. Include avocados, nuts, seeds, and olive oil in your diet as sources of healthful fats.

It is critical to balance macronutrients since it:

Promotes Satiety: A well-balanced diet of carbs, proteins, and fats can keep you feeling fuller for longer, lowering your chances of overeating.

Carbohydrates give immediate energy, but lipids provide continuous energy. Protein aids in the repair and construction of tissues, which is essential for an active lifestyle.

Increases Nutrient Intake: A well-balanced diet contains a wide variety of vital nutrients, ensuring that your body receives what it requires for optimal operation.

To establish macronutrient balance, follow these steps:

Incorporate items from all dietary categories into your diet.

Consider your personal nutritional needs, such as those of athletes, vegans, or people with unique health issues.

To ensure you fulfill your macronutrient targets, keep a meal journal or use nutrition apps to track your macronutrient consumption.

3. Individualization:

It is critical to tailor portion sizes and macronutrient ratios to your specific requirements and goals. A diet that works for one person may not work for another. Age, gender, exercise level, and health issues are all factors in establishing your nutritional requirements.

Healthy Eating Habits for Long-Term Success

Healthy eating habits lay the groundwork for long-term improvements in your health, fitness, and general well-being. While there is no one-size-fits-all solution to healthy eating, some practices can assist you in developing a balanced and long-term relationship with food. Here are some essential healthy eating practices for long-term success:

1. **Consume a Well-balanced Diet:** Aim for a macronutrient (carbohydrates, proteins, and fats) and micronutrient (vitamins and minerals) balance. This ensures that you acquire a diverse spectrum of critical nutrients.

2. **Portion Management:** To avoid overeating, pay attention to portion proportions. To aid with portion management, use smaller plates, bowls, and utensils.

3. **Mindfulness in Eating:** Eat mindfully, appreciating every mouthful and paying attention to hunger and fullness signs. While eating, avoid distractions such as devices.

4. **Hydration:** Drink plenty of water throughout the day to stay hydrated. Thirst is sometimes confused with hunger.

5. **Consume Whole Foods:** Fruits, vegetables, whole grains, lean meats, and healthy fats should be prioritized as whole, unprocessed foods. These foods are high in nutrients and promote general wellness.

6. Diet High in Fiber: Include fiber-rich meals to aid digestion and enhance fullness. Fruits, vegetables, legumes, and whole grains are all high in fiber.

7. Macronutrients in Balance: In your meals, aim for a balance of carbs, proteins, and fats. This aids in the regulation of energy levels and the control of hunger.

8. Good Fats: Include avocados, nuts, seeds, and olive oil in your diet as sources of healthful fats. Healthy fats are beneficial to brain function and nutrition absorption.

9. Proteins that are low in fat: Choose lean protein sources such as chicken, fish, tofu, legumes, and low-fat dairy. Protein is necessary for muscle maintenance as well as general health.

10. Restrict Added Sugars: Reduce your intake of added sugars and sugary beverages, which can cause energy spikes and crashes.

11. Schedule Meals and Snacks: Plan your meals and snacks ahead of time to ensure you have healthy alternatives on hand. When you're hungry, this decreases the temptation to make less healthful choices.

12 Cooking at Home: When feasible, prepare homemade meals since you have more control over the ingredients and cooking processes.

13. Mindful Eating: Consider emotional eating triggers and attempt to distinguish between actual hunger and emotional desires.

14. Be adaptable: Allow yourself to indulge in occasional snacks or meals that may not fit into your usual healthy eating regimen. Flexibility fosters a long-term connection with food.

15. Pay Attention to Your Body: Pay attention to your body's hunger and fullness signals. Eat only when you're hungry and quit when you're full.

16. Maintain Your Knowledge: Maintain your dietary knowledge by reading reputable sources and receiving advice from qualified dietitians or nutritionists as required.

17. Stay away from extreme diets: Avoid excessive diets that promise quick results. These are frequently unsustainable and can result in health problems.

18. Set attainable goals: Set attainable and attainable health and fitness objectives. Small, incremental modifications are more likely to result in long-term success.

19. Seek Help: Consider obtaining the advice of a healthcare practitioner or a qualified dietitian if you have specific dietary objectives or health issues. They can give tailored advice.

CHAPTER 4

MEAL PLANNING AND RECIPES

Weekly Meal Planning for Endomorphs

Meal planning is an effective strategy for endomorphs (or anyone) looking to manage their weight and achieve their nutritional goals. It helps you make healthier food choices, control portion sizes, and maintain a balanced diet. Here's a weekly meal planning guide tailored to endomorphs:

Week 1

Day 1:

Breakfast:

Scrambled eggs with spinach and tomatoes.

Whole-grain toast.

A serving of berries.

Lunch: Grilled chicken breast salad with mixed greens, cucumbers, and a vinaigrette dressing.

Quinoa on the side.

Snack: Greek yogurt with a drizzle of honey and a handful of almonds.

Dinner:

Baked salmon with a lemon-dill sauce.

Steamed broccoli.

Brown rice.

Day 2:

Breakfast:

Oatmeal topped with sliced bananas and chopped walnuts.

A glass of unsweetened almond milk.

Lunch:

Lentil soup.

A mixed greens salad with cherry tomatoes and a balsamic vinaigrette dressing.

Snack:

Sliced cucumbers and hummus.

Dinner:

Stir-fried tofu with mixed vegetables in a ginger-soy sauce.

Quinoa.

Day 3:

Breakfast:

Greek yogurt parfait with granola and fresh berries.

Lunch:

Turkey and avocado wrap with whole-grain tortilla.

Mixed greens salad.

Snack:

Carrot sticks and sliced bell peppers with a light dip.

Dinner:

Grilled lean beef steak.

Roasted sweet potatoes.

Steamed green beans.

Day 4:

Breakfast:

Whole-grain waffles with a dollop of Greek yogurt and sliced strawberries.

Lunch:

Chickpea and vegetable curry.

Brown rice.

Snack:

A small apple with almond butter.

Dinner:

Baked chicken breast with rosemary and garlic.

Sauteed spinach.

Quinoa.

Day 5:

Breakfast:

Smoothie with spinach, banana, protein powder, and almond milk.

Lunch:

Mixed bean salad with black beans, kidney beans, corn, and a lime-cilantro dressing.

Snack:

Cottage cheese with pineapple chunks.

Dinner:

Grilled shrimp skewers with a side of roasted Brussels sprouts.

Quinoa.

Day 6:

Breakfast:

Vegetable omelet with mushrooms, bell peppers, and onions.

Whole-grain toast.

Lunch:

Turkey and vegetable stir-fry with a light teriyaki sauce.

Brown rice.

Snack:

A handful of mixed nuts.

Dinner:

Baked cod with tomato and olive salsa.

Steamed asparagus.

Quinoa.

Day 7:

Breakfast:

Whole-grain pancakes with a drizzle of maple syrup and a side of mixed berries.

Lunch: Quinoa salad with chickpeas, cucumber, and a lemon-tahini dressing.

Snack:

Sliced apple with a sprinkle of cinnamon.

Dinner:

Grilled lean pork chops.

Roasted butternut squash.

Steamed broccoli.

Week 2

Day 1:

Breakfast:

Scrambled eggs with sautéed spinach and mushrooms.

Whole-grain toast with avocado spread.

A side of mixed berries.

Lunch:

Grilled chicken breast with a lemon-herb marinade.

Quinoa and roasted vegetable salad.

A small serving of Greek yogurt.

Snack:

Sliced cucumbers and cherry tomatoes with hummus.

Dinner: Baked tilapia with a garlic-lime marinade.

Steamed broccoli and cauliflower.

Brown rice.

Day 2:

Breakfast:

Greek yogurt parfait with granola, sliced peaches, and a drizzle of honey.

Lunch:

Lentil and vegetable stir-fry with tofu.

A mixed greens salad with balsamic vinaigrette dressing.

Snack:

A handful of mixed nuts and dried cranberries.

Dinner:

Baked turkey meatballs with marinara sauce.

Zucchini noodles.

A side of steamed green beans.

Day 3:

Breakfast:

Smoothie with spinach, banana, almond milk, and a scoop of protein powder.

Lunch:

Chickpea and quinoa salad with diced cucumber, red onion, and a lemon-tahini dressing.

Snack:

Sliced bell peppers and baby carrots with guacamole.

Dinner:

Grilled lean beef kebabs with bell peppers and onions.

Quinoa cooked with diced tomatoes and herbs.

Day 4:

Breakfast:

Whole-grain waffles with a dollop of cottage cheese and mixed berries.

Lunch:

Black bean and vegetable chili.

A small mixed greens salad with a light vinaigrette.

Snack:

Sliced pear with almond butter.

Dinner:

Baked salmon with a honey-mustard glaze.

Roasted Brussels sprouts.

Quinoa.

Day 5:

Breakfast:

Scrambled eggs with diced tomatoes and feta cheese.

Whole-grain toast.

Lunch:

Turkey and avocado salad with mixed greens, cherry tomatoes, and a creamy dressing.

Snack:

A small serving of cottage cheese with pineapple chunks.

Dinner:

Grilled shrimp and vegetable skewers with a lemon-herb marinade.

Brown rice.

Day 6:

Breakfast:

Whole-grain oatmeal with sliced bananas and chopped pecans.

Lunch: Quinoa and chickpea bowl with roasted butternut squash, arugula, and a tahini dressing.

Snack:

Sliced apple with a sprinkle of cinnamon and a side of Greek yogurt.

Dinner:

Grilled lean pork tenderloin with a balsamic glaze.

Steamed asparagus and carrots.

Brown rice.

Day 7:

Breakfast:

Whole-grain pancakes with fresh blueberries and a drizzle of pure maple syrup.

Lunch:

Mixed bean and vegetable soup.

A side salad with mixed greens and a light vinaigrette.

Snack:

Sliced cucumber and baby carrots with tzatziki sauce.

Dinner:

Baked chicken breast with a tomato-basil topping.

Roasted sweet potatoes.

Steamed green beans.

Breakfast Recipes

1. A parfait of Greek yogurt

Ingredients:

Greek yogurt, one cup

Fresh berries, such as strawberries, blueberries, and raspberries, to the tune of 1/2 cup

1/4 cup of cereal

1 teaspoon of honey

Instructions:

Half of the Greek yogurt should be layered in a glass or dish.

On top, sprinkle with half the berries and half the granola.

Add honey to the dish.

With the remaining ingredients, repeat the stacking procedure.

Serve right away and delight in!

Approximate Nutritional Data

300 calories

15g of protein

45g of carbohydrates

5g of fiber

Fat: 8g

2. Breakfast Quesadilla with Spinach and Mushroom

Ingredients:

2 substantial whole-wheat tortillas

4 big, beaten eggs

baby spinach leaves, 1 cup

Sliced mushrooms in a cup

1/4 cup of cheddar cheese, shredded

pepper and salt as desired

Olive oil or cooking spray for the pan

Instructions:

Cooking spray or olive oil should be sparingly applied to a non-stick pan before heating it over medium heat.

Sliced mushrooms should be added and sautéed until they begin to brown.

Sauté until baby spinach has wilted after adding.

The eggs should be added to the pan with the veggies and scrambled until fully done.

One tortilla should be placed in the skillet along with half of the egg and veggie mixture and half of the cheese.

Place the second tortilla on top and gently push it down.

Cook the tortilla until it is crispy and the cheese has melted, about 2-3 minutes on each side.

Serve after cooling down and slicing.

Approximate Nutritional Data

340 calories

18g of protein

30g of carbohydrates

5g of fiber

Fat: 16g

3. Chia Seed Pudding made over night

Ingredients: Chia seeds, 2 teaspoons

(Or any other milk of your choosing) 1/2 cup of unsweetened almond milk

One-half teaspoon of vanilla extract

1 tablespoon maple syrup or honey (optional)

For the topping, use fresh fruit (such as sliced bananas or berries).

Instructions: Chia seeds, almond milk, vanilla extract, and honey (if used) should all be combined in a jar or other container.

Make sure there are no clumps and stir thoroughly.

Refrigerate overnight (or at least for two to three hours) after sealing the container.

Give it a nice stir in the morning, then top it with fresh fruit and eat!

Approximate Nutritional Data

180 calories

4g. protein

23g of carbohydrates

9g of fiber

Fat: 8g

4 Vegetable Omelette

Ingredients: two huge eggs

14 cups of bell peppers, diced

tomato dice, one-fourth cup

1/fourth cup minced spinach 1/fourth cup diced onions

pepper and salt as desired

Olive oil or cooking spray for the pan

Instructions:

In a bowl, beat the eggs well.

Cooking spray or olive oil should be sparingly applied to a non-stick pan before heating it over medium heat.

To the skillet, add tomatoes, bell peppers, and onions. When they begin to soften, sauté.

Sauté the spinach until wilted after adding it.

Add salt and pepper, then pour the beaten eggs over the veggies and heat until the edges begin to set.

Then, carefully fold it in half and cook it for one more minute, or until it is completely set.

Slice it, then place it on a dish and serve.

Approximate Nutritional Data

200 calories

12g of protein

9g of carbohydrates

2g of fiber

Fat: 14g

5. Smoothie with peanut butter and banana

Ingredients:

one ripe banana

2 tablespoons of unsweetened peanut butter

1 cup almond milk without sugar (or any other milk of your choosing)

Oats, rolled, 14 cup

One teaspoon of optional honey

Ice cubes, if desired

Instructions:

Blend the items in a blender.

Blend till creamy and smooth.

If you like a cooler smoothie, add ice cubes.

Pour into a glass, then sip.

Approximate Nutritional Data

350 calories

9g protein

40g of carbohydrates

5g of fiber

Fat: 19g

Lunch Recipes

1. Quinoa with grilled chicken salad

Ingredients:

grilled chicken breast, sliced, 4 ounces (113 grams)

cooked quinoa, 1 cup

2 cups of greens, mixed

Half a cup of cherry tomatoes

14 cups of cucumber slices

Balsamic vinaigrette dressing, two teaspoons

Instructions:

The mixed greens, quinoa, cherry tomatoes, and cucumber should all be combined in a big dish.

Add balsamic vinaigrette dressing and drizzle, then toss to coat.

Add grilled chicken pieces on top.

Dispense and savor!

Approximate Nutritional Data

400 calories

30g of protein

35g of carbohydrates

5g of fiber

Fat: 15g

2. Avocado and Chickpea Wrap

Ingredients:

one whole-wheat tortilla

1/2 cup mashed chickpeas

sliced avocado, half

1/4 cup red bell peppers, chopped

14 cups of chopped lettuce

Spreading hummus is optional.

Instructions:

If used, lay the tortilla flat and distribute the hummus evenly.

Add sliced red bell pepper, shredded lettuce, avocado slices, and mashed chickpeas.

The tortilla should be rolled up, divided in half, and sometimes fastened with toothpicks.

Dispense and savor!

Approximate Nutritional Data

350 calories

10g of protein

50g of carbohydrates

12g of fiber

Fat: 14g

3. Bowl of quinoa and black beans

Ingredients:

cooked quinoa, 1 cup

1/2 cup cooked or canned black beans

1/4 cup fresh, frozen, or canned corn kernels

1/4 cup red onion, chopped

1/4 cup red bell peppers, chopped

Salsa, two tablespoons

Fresh cilantro can be used as a garnish.

Instructions:

Cooked quinoa, black beans, corn, red onion, and red bell pepper should all be combined in a dish.

Add salsa and stir to combine.

If desired, add some fresh cilantro as a garnish.

Dispense and savor!

Approximate Nutritional Data

350 calories

13g of protein

64g of carbohydrates

11g of fiber

Fat: 3g

4. Salad with Turkey and Avocado

Ingredients:

113g of sliced turkey breast, 4 oz.

Sliced half an avocado, two cups of mixed greens

Half a cup of cherry tomatoes

14 cups of cucumber slices

Drizzling balsamic vinaigrette dressing

Instructions:

On a dish, arrange the mixed greens.

Slices of turkey, avocado, cherry tomatoes, and cucumber are added on top.

Add a balsamic vinaigrette dressing drizzle.

Dispense and savor!

Approximate Nutritional Data

320 calories

20g of protein

20g of carbohydrates

8g of fiber

Fat: 20g

5. Vegetable and Lentil Soup

Ingredients:

cooked lentils, 1 cup

1 cup chopped mixed veggies, including bell peppers, carrots, and celery

onions, diced, in a cup

1 minced garlic clove

4 cups of veggie broth

1/9 cup olive oil

pepper and salt as desired

Instructions:

In a soup pot, warm up the olive oil over medium heat.

Add minced garlic and chopped onions. until fragrant, sauté.

Cook for a few minutes after adding the diced veggies.

The veggie broth should be added and brought to a boil.

When the veggies are ready, add the cooked lentils and turn the heat down.

Add salt and pepper to taste.

Serve warm.

Approximate Nutritional Data

250 calories

14g of protein

46g of carbohydrates

14g of fiber

Fat: 2g

6. Lettuce wraps with tuna salad

Ingredients: 1 can (5 oz) of drained tuna in water

Greek yogurt (or mayonnaise) in two teaspoons

1/9 cup Dijon mustard

14 cups of celery, chopped

1/4 cup red onion, chopped

lettuce leaves (such as Romaine or Iceberg) for wrapping

Instructions: Tuna, Greek yogurt (or mayonnaise), Dijon mustard, sliced celery, and diced red onion should all be combined in a dish.

Fill lettuce leaves with the tuna salad mixture with a spoon.

The lettuce leaves should be rolled up and, if necessary, secured with toothpicks.

Dispense and savor!

Approximate Nutritional Data

230 calories

27g of protein

7g of carbohydrates

2g of fiber

Fat: 10g

7. Hummus with vegetable Wrap

Ingredients: one whole-wheat tortilla

two teaspoons of hummus

cucumber slices

red bell peppers, sliced

sliced avocado with carrot

brand-new spinach leaves

Instructions:

Over the whole-wheat tortilla, evenly spread hummus.

On top of the hummus, arrange the cucumber, red bell pepper, carrot, avocado, and spinach leaves.

The tortilla should be rolled up, divided in half, and sometimes fastened with toothpicks.

Dispense and savor!

Approximate Nutritional Data

290 calories

7g protein

35g of carbohydrates

10g of fiber

Fat: 14g

Dinner Recipes

1. Baked Lemon Herb Salmon

Ingredients:

6 oz (170g) salmon fillet

1 tablespoon olive oil

Juice of 1 lemon

1 teaspoon dried herbs (such as thyme, rosemary, or dill)

Salt and pepper to taste

Instructions:

Preheat the oven to 400°F (200°C).

Place the salmon fillet on a baking sheet lined with parchment paper.

Drizzle with olive oil and lemon juice.

Sprinkle with dried herbs, salt, and pepper.

Bake for about 15-20 minutes or until the salmon flakes easily with a fork.

Serve with steamed vegetables and quinoa.

Nutritional Information (approx.):

Calories: 300

Protein: 25g

Carbohydrates: 0g

Fiber: 0g

Fat: 22g

2. Grilled Chicken with Roasted Vegetables

Ingredients:

4 oz (113g) grilled chicken breast

Assorted vegetables (bell peppers, zucchini, broccoli, carrots)

1 tablespoon olive oil

Salt, pepper, and herbs for seasoning

Instructions:

Preheat the grill or grill pan.

Toss the vegetables with olive oil, salt, pepper, and herbs.

Grill the chicken until cooked through, about 6-8 minutes per side.

Meanwhile, roast the vegetables in the oven at 400°F (200°C) for 20-25 minutes.

Serve the grilled chicken with roasted vegetables.

Nutritional Information (approx.):

Calories: 350

Protein: 30g

Carbohydrates: 10g

Fiber: 4g

Fat: 20g

3. Quinoa Stuffed Bell Peppers

Ingredients:

2 bell peppers, halved and seeds removed

1 cup cooked quinoa

1/2 cup black beans, drained and rinsed

1/2 cup diced tomatoes

1/4 cup diced onion

1/4 cup shredded cheese (cheddar, mozzarella, or your choice)

1 teaspoon chili powder

Salt and pepper to taste

Instructions:

Preheat the oven to 375°F (190°C).

In a bowl, mix cooked quinoa, black beans, diced tomatoes, diced onion, chili powder, salt, and pepper.

Fill the halved bell peppers with the quinoa mixture.

Sprinkle shredded cheese on top.

Place the stuffed peppers on a baking sheet and bake for about 20-25 minutes.

Serve with a side salad.

Nutritional Information (approx.):

Calories: 300

Protein: 12g

Carbohydrates: 45g

Fiber: 10g

Fat: 10g

4. Vegetable Stir-Fry with Tofu

Ingredients:

4 oz (113g) tofu, cubed

Assorted vegetables (broccoli, bell peppers, snap peas, carrots)

2 tablespoons soy sauce

1 tablespoon sesame oil

1 teaspoon minced garlic

1 teaspoon minced ginger

Red pepper flakes (optional)

Sesame seeds for garnish

Instructions:

Heat sesame oil in a wok or skillet over medium-high heat.

Add minced garlic and ginger, and sauté for a minute.

Add tofu cubes and cook until golden brown.

Add assorted vegetables and stir-fry until tender-crisp.

Drizzle with soy sauce and red pepper flakes if desired.

Serve over brown rice or quinoa, garnished with sesame seeds.

Nutritional Information (approx.):

Calories: 320

Protein: 15g

Carbohydrates: 25g

Fiber: 7g

Fat: 20g

5. Turkey and Vegetable Skillet

Ingredients:

4 oz (113g) ground turkey

Assorted vegetables (zucchini, bell peppers, onions)

1 teaspoon olive oil

1 teaspoon chili powder

1/2 teaspoon cumin

Salt and pepper to taste

Whole-grain tortillas for serving

Instructions:

Heat olive oil in a skillet over medium heat.

Add ground turkey and cook until browned.

Add diced vegetables and cook until tender.

Season with chili powder, cumin, salt, and pepper.

Serve the turkey and vegetable mixture with whole-grain tortillas for wrapping.

Nutritional Information (approx.):

Calories: 300

Protein: 20g

Carbohydrates: 25g

Fiber: 6g

Fat: 15g

6. Baked Eggplant Parmesan

Ingredients:

1 medium eggplant, sliced into rounds

1 cup marinara sauce (low-sodium)

1/2 cup part-skim mozzarella cheese, shredded

2 tablespoons grated Parmesan cheese

1/4 cup whole-wheat breadcrumbs

Fresh basil leaves for garnish

Instructions:

Preheat the oven to 375°F (190°C).

Lightly coat eggplant slices with olive oil and arrange them on a baking sheet.

Bake for about 20 minutes or until tender.

In a baking dish, layer marinara sauce, eggplant slices, mozzarella cheese, and Parmesan cheese.

Repeat the layers and top with breadcrumbs.

Bake for an additional 20-25 minutes or until bubbly and golden.

Garnish with fresh basil leaves before serving.

Nutritional Information (approx.):

Calories: 250

Protein: 10g

Carbohydrates: 30g

Fiber: 10g

Fat: 10g

7. Lentil and Vegetable Curry

Ingredients: 1 cup cooked lentils

Assorted vegetables (bell peppers, carrots, peas, potatoes)

1 cup canned diced tomatoes

1 cup light coconut milk

1 tablespoon curry powder

1 teaspoon minced garlic

1 teaspoon minced ginger

Salt and pepper to taste

Fresh cilantro for garnish

Instructions: In a large pot, heat a little oil over medium heat.

Add minced garlic and ginger, and sauté for a minute.

Add assorted vegetables and cook until slightly softened.

Stir in curry powder, canned diced tomatoes, and cooked lentils.

Pour in light coconut milk and simmer until vegetables are tender.

Season with salt and pepper.

Garnish with fresh cilantro before serving.

Serve with brown rice or whole-grain naan.

Nutritional Information (approx.):

Calories: 320

Protein: 15g

Carbohydrates: 45g

Fiber: 12g

Fat: 6g

8. Sweet Potato and Black Bean Quesadillas

Ingredients:

2 whole-grain tortillas

1 cup mashed sweet potatoes

1/2 cup black beans, drained and rinsed

1/4 cup diced red onion

1/4 cup diced red bell pepper

1/2 teaspoon cumin

1/2 teaspoon chili powder

Salt and pepper to taste

Instructions:

Spread mashed sweet potatoes evenly on one side of each tortilla.

Sprinkle black beans, diced red onion, diced red bell pepper, cumin, chili powder, salt, and pepper on top.

Fold the tortillas in half.

Heat a skillet over medium-high heat and lightly coat with cooking spray or olive oil.

Cook quesadillas for 2-3 minutes on each side or until crispy.

Slice and serve with salsa or Greek yogurt.

Nutritional Information (approx.):

Calories: 350

Protein: 12g

Carbohydrates: 60g

Fiber: 12g

Fat: 7g

9. Stir-Fried Shrimp with Vegetables

Ingredients:

4 oz (113g) shrimp, peeled and deveined

Assorted vegetables (broccoli, snap peas, bell peppers, carrots)

1 tablespoon soy sauce

1 tablespoon hoisin sauce

1 teaspoon minced garlic

1 teaspoon minced ginger

1 teaspoon sesame oil

Red pepper flakes (optional)

Cooked brown rice for serving

Instructions:

In a bowl, combine soy sauce, hoisin sauce, minced garlic, minced ginger, and red pepper flakes (if desired).

Heat sesame oil in a wok or skillet over medium-high heat.

Add shrimp and stir-fry until pink and opaque.

Add assorted vegetables and continue to stir-fry until tender-crisp.

Pour the sauce mixture over the shrimp and vegetables, and stir to coat.

Serve over cooked brown rice.

Nutritional Information (approx.):

Calories: 320

Protein: 25g

Carbohydrates: 40g

Fiber: 6g

Fat: 6g

10. Veggie and Chickpea Curry

Ingredients:

1 cup cooked chickpeas (canned or cooked)

Assorted vegetables (cauliflower, bell peppers, peas, onions)

1 cup canned diced tomatoes

1 cup light coconut milk

1 tablespoon curry powder

1 teaspoon minced garlic

1 teaspoon minced ginger

Salt and pepper to taste

Fresh cilantro for garnish

Instructions:

In a large pot, heat a little oil over medium heat.

Add minced garlic and ginger, and sauté for a minute.

Add assorted vegetables and cook until slightly softened.

Stir in curry powder, canned diced tomatoes, cooked chickpeas, and light coconut milk.

Simmer until vegetables are tender and the curry thickens.

Season with salt and pepper.

Garnish with fresh cilantro before serving.

Serve with brown rice or whole-grain naan.

Nutritional Information (approx.):

Calories: 320

Protein: 14g

Carbohydrates: 45g

Fiber: 12g

Fat: 6g

Tips for Dining Out and Social Events

When you're attempting to maintain a balanced diet and make smart food choices, eating out and attending social events can be difficult. However, with some careful preparation and decision-making, you may still enjoy these occasions while staying on track with your nutritional objectives. Here are some pointers for dining out and socializing:

1. Plan ahead of time:

Check the Menu Ahead of Time: If feasible, go through the restaurant's menu online before you go. Look for healthier alternatives and organize your meals ahead of time.

Eat a Small Snack: Before heading out, have a small, balanced snack to help control your appetite and prevent overeating.

2. Make Sound Decisions:

Choose lean protein choices such as chicken, fish, or tofu that can be grilled, roasted, or steamed.

Order salads or vegetable-based dishes as sides or main courses to enhance your fiber intake.

Portion Control: Watch your portion sizes. Consider splitting an entree with a buddy or ordering a to-go box to take home half of your meal before you begin eating.

Avoid options that are fried or creamy: Deep-fried and creamy foods should be avoided since they are heavy in calories and saturated fats.

Instead of sugary soft drinks, choose water, herbal tea, or other low-calorie liquids.

3. Personalize Your Order:

Don't be afraid to tailor your order to your nutritional needs. choose dressings and sauces on the side, or choose grilled rather than fried dishes.

4. Be Wary of Drinks: Limit Alcohol Consumption: If you prefer to drink alcohol, do so in moderation. Alcohol can increase calorie intake and lessen inhibitions, resulting in bad eating choices.

Stay hydrated by drinking water during the meal to help limit your appetite.

5. Exercise Portion Control: Use Smaller Plates: To assist reduce portion sizes during social gatherings featuring buffets or finger appetizers, use a smaller plate.

Pay Attention to Your Hunger: Take note of your body's hunger signs. Eat gently and end when you're satisfied but not stuffed.

6. Social Assistance: Share Your objectives: Inform your friends and family about your dietary objectives and solicit their assistance in selecting restaurants and foods that meet your requirements.

7. Mindfulness in Eating: Savor Every Bite: Take your time with your food. Eating slowly might assist you in recognizing when you are full.

Stay Present: Instead of focusing primarily on the meal, engage in conversations and social interactions.

8. Desserts and Snacks:

Desserts should be shared: If you desire dessert, consider splitting it with someone to enjoy a lesser piece.

Choose Wisely: If available, look for fruit-based or lower-calorie dessert alternatives.

9. Exercise Moderation:

It is acceptable to indulge on occasion, but moderation is essential. You don't have to give up all of your favorite foods or snacks; simply eat them in smaller portions and less frequently.

10. For Social Events:

Bring a Healthy Dish: If you're going to a potluck or party, bring a healthy dish that you love to guarantee there's something nutritional accessible.

Be Courteous but Firm: Politely deny food or beverages that do not correspond to your dietary objectives. You may say, "No thank you, I'm trying to eat healthier."

CHAPTER 5

EXERCISE FOR ENDOMORPHS

Exercise's Role in Endomorph Weight Management

Exercise is essential for endomorph weight control. Endomorphs have a natural propensity to accumulate fat and may find it more difficult to shed weight or maintain a healthy weight than other body types. Regular physical exercise, on the other hand, may be a tremendous tool for endomorphs in terms of weight management, overall health, and accomplishing fitness objectives. Here's how exercise helps endomorph weight management:

1. Improves Metabolism:

Exercise, especially strength training and high-intensity interval training (HIIT), can boost metabolism. A faster metabolic rate indicates that the body burns more calories at rest, making weight management simpler.

2. Calories Burned:

Physical activity burns calories, whether it's cardiovascular exercise like jogging or strength training routines like weightlifting. This calorie expenditure helps with weight reduction or maintenance.

3. Increases Muscle Mass:

Endomorphs must build and retain lean muscle mass through resistance exercise. Because muscle burns more calories than fat at rest, increasing muscle mass can aid in long-term weight management.

4. Aids in Fat Loss:

Regular exercise, particularly cardiovascular workouts, aids the body's ability to burn stored fat for energy. This might result in a decrease in total body fat percentage.

5. Controls Insulin Sensitivity:

Exercise promotes insulin sensitivity, allowing the body to better control blood sugar levels. Improved blood sugar management can help avoid extra fat storage and lower the risk of type 2 diabetes.

6. Increases Energy Consumption:

Physical exercise boosts daily energy expenditure, which contributes to the calorie deficit required for weight loss.

This is especially crucial for endomorphs, who are prone to gaining weight.

7. Better Cardiovascular Health:

Aerobic activity, such as jogging, cycling, or swimming regularly, can enhance cardiovascular health and lower the risk of heart disease, which is critical for general well-being.

8. Aids in Appetite Regulation:

Exercise can assist in the regulation of hunger hormones, making it simpler to manage food desires and quantity management.

9. It improves mood and motivation: Endorphins are released during exercise, which might improve mood and motivation. This is especially beneficial for endomorphs who may confront mental obstacles in their weight-loss quest.

10. Boosts Long-Term Weight Maintenance:

Incorporating exercise into your daily routine not only aids in weight reduction but also raises the chance of long-term weight loss maintenance.

11. Supports a Healthy Lifestyle:

A healthy lifestyle begins with regular exercise. It promotes not just weight loss but also physical and emotional wellbeing.

As an endomorph, it's critical to include a mix of aerobic, strength, and flexibility workouts in your fitness program for optimal weight control. Furthermore, consistency is essential. Make exercise a habit, and consider working with a fitness expert or nutritionist to develop a personalized exercise and nutrition plan suited to your unique objectives and needs. While exercise is important, a healthy diet and general lifestyle choices are also important components of good weight management.

Creating an Endomorph Exercise Program

Endomorph exercise programs should include a combination of aerobic activity, strength training, and flexibility work. The objective is to increase metabolism, lean muscle mass, and fat reduction. Here's a step-by-step method for creating an endomorph-specific fitness program:

1. Determine Your Fitness Level: Assess your current fitness level before you begin. This will assist you in setting realistic objectives and determining the intensity of your workouts.

2. Establish Specific Objectives: Define explicit, quantifiable, and attainable objectives. Having specific objectives can lead your workout regimen, whether it's weight reduction, muscle gain, or enhanced cardiovascular health.

3. Combine Cardiovascular and Strength Training: Cardiovascular workouts (cardio) and strength training are both part of a well-rounded program.

Aim for at least 150 minutes of moderate-intensity cardio per week or 75 minutes of vigorous-intensity cardio per week. Brisk walking, running, cycling, swimming, or dancing are all options. Cardiovascular exercise burns calories and improves heart health.

Strength Training: Include strength training activities at least twice a week. Squats, deadlifts, bench presses, and pull-ups are examples of complex exercises that train numerous muscular groups. Lean muscular mass increases metabolism and assists in fat reduction.

4. High-Intensity Interval Training (HIIT) and Circuit Training: Consider incorporating circuit training or high-intensity interval training into your workout program. These routines are effective at burning calories and increasing fat reduction. They consist of short bursts of high-intensity exercise followed by short rest intervals.

5. Concentrate on Core Strength: Endomorphs may have a propensity to retain fat in the abdomen. Core strengthening activities such as planks, Russian twists, and leg lifts can assist tone and tightening this area.

6. Include Work Flexibility and Mobility: Stretching and mobility exercises should be done regularly to increase flexibility and avoid injuries. Yoga and Pilates lessons are great for endomorphs because they increase flexibility and body awareness.

7. Put Consistency First: Consistency is essential for reaching and sustaining fitness objectives. To stay motivated, make fitness a regular part of your routine and pick things that you like.

8. Track Progress: To measure your improvement, keep a workout log or utilize fitness monitoring apps. Tracking your exercises, weight, body measurements, and other pertinent data will help you remain on track and make required program modifications.

9. Hydration and nutrition: Exercise by itself is insufficient for good weight management. Maintain a healthy diet and remain hydrated. A healthy diet that supports your exercise objectives is essential.

10. Rest and Recovery: After each workout, give your body time to recuperate. Adequate rest is critical for muscle recovery and general health.

11. Seek Professional Help: Consider working with a licensed personal trainer or fitness expert if you are new to training or have special fitness objectives. They can assist you in developing a program that is suited to your specific requirements.

12. Be Patient:

Keep in mind that growth takes time. Be patient and persistent in your efforts, and don't let little failures discourage you.

Endomorph Cardiovascular Workouts

Cardiovascular workouts are an essential part of an endomorph fitness routine. These routines help you burn calories, boost your cardiovascular health, and lose weight. Here are some efficient cardiovascular routines designed specifically for endomorphs:

Walking briskly: Brisk walking is a low-impact cardiovascular workout that most individuals can do. It's a great option for novices and people who want to ease into a training regimen.

On most days of the week, aim for at least 30 minutes of brisk walking. As your fitness level increases, gradually increase the time and intensity.

Running or jogging: Jogging or running is a more intense kind of cardiovascular exercise. It can assist you in losing weight and improving your cardiovascular fitness.

If you're new to running, start with a run-walk method. Aim for longer continuous runs as your stamina develops.

To increase calorie burn, include interval training by alternating between intervals of quicker running and slower recovery jogging.

Cycling: Cycling, whether on a stationary bike or outside, is an efficient technique to exercise your leg muscles and raise your heart rate.

Interval training may be used by riding at a high effort for brief bursts, followed by recovery periods at a reduced level.

Swimming: Swimming is a low-impact cardiovascular activity that works the entire body. It's easy on the joints and perfect for endomorphs who are concerned about joint impact.

To enhance calorie burn, swim laps at a moderate to strenuous speed.

Dancing: Workouts focused on dance, such as Zumba or dance aerobics, are a fun and efficient approach to raising your heart rate.

These workouts can help you increase your cardiovascular endurance while also allowing you to express yourself through dance.

Elliptical Machine: A low-impact, full-body exercise on an elliptical machine is gentle on the joints.

You may enhance the intensity of your workout by adjusting the resistance and incline.

Climbing the Stairs: Climbing steps, whether on a stair climber machine or real stairs, is a great method to work your leg muscles and raise your heart rate.

It is a high-intensity activity that can help you burn calories and improve your cardiovascular fitness.

HIIT (High-Intensity Interval Training): HIIT exercises consist of short bursts of high-intensity activity followed by short rest intervals. This method can be quite helpful for losing weight and boosting cardiovascular fitness.

HIIT may be used for a variety of aerobic workouts, including sprinting, cycling, and bodyweight exercises like burpees and jumping jacks.

Group Exercise Classes: Participating in group exercise courses such as spinning, kickboxing, or aerobics may help to diversify your cardio regimen while also encouraging social dynamics.

Outdoor Recreation: Participate in outdoor activities such as hiking, trail jogging, or sports such as tennis or basketball. These exercises can give both cardiovascular and recreational advantages.

Muscle Tone Through Strength Training

Strength training is a vital component of any fitness regimen that aims to increase muscle tone and achieve a sculpted body. Muscle tone refers to the firmness and definition of your muscles, which may be achieved by strength training by increasing muscle mass and decreasing body fat. Here's how to design a muscle tone strength training program:

1. Establish Your Objectives: Define your precise muscle tone objectives. Do you want to tone your complete body or just certain muscle areas, such as your arms, legs, or core? Having specific goals can assist you in creating an efficient fitness regimen.

2. Select the Appropriate Exercises: Include a variety of compound and isolation workouts. Compound exercises, including squats, deadlifts, and bench presses, engage many muscle groups at the same time and are extremely effective for increasing total muscular tone. Isolation workouts, such as bicep curls and leg extensions, target certain muscles and can help define them.

3. Create a Split Routine: To achieve balanced development and recuperation, divide your strength training routines into different muscle groups or body regions. Working on separate muscle parts on different days, such as the legs, chest, back, and arms, is a frequent split program.

4. Repetition and Resistance: For each exercise, select the proper amount of resistance. You should be able to finish your repetitions while maintaining proper form but yet feeling pushed.

2-4 sets of 8-15 repetitions for each exercise are ideal. Higher repetitions with modest weights can aid in the development of muscular endurance and tone.

5. Gradual Overload: As your strength and endurance develop, gradually increase the resistance (weights) or repetitions. This gradual stress is necessary for muscular development and tone.

6. Complete Range of Motion: To properly engage the target muscles, do each exercise over its whole range of motion. To lift weights, avoid utilizing momentum or swinging.

7. Rest and recuperation: Allow enough time between sets and muscle groups. Muscles require rest and growth time.

Allow at least 48 hours between training the same muscle group again.

8. Include Core Exercises: A strong core is necessary for good muscular tone and stability. Include workouts that target your core muscles, such as planks, Russian twists, and leg lifts.

9. Combine cardiovascular and strength training: Combining aerobic and strength training sessions can help reduce total body fat and show the toned muscles beneath.

10. Proper Nutrition: Feed your body a well-balanced diet rich in protein to help muscle repair and development. Make sure you're getting enough calories to sustain your level of exercise and muscle-building goals.

11. Consistency: Consistency is essential for improving muscular tone. Maintain your strength training regimen and gradually push your muscles.

12. Form and Technique: To avoid injury and optimize results, maintain good form and technique during each exercise. If you're new to strength training or want to guarantee perfect form, consider working with a certified personal trainer.

13. Flexibility and Mobility: Include stretching and mobility exercises in your regimen to increase flexibility and decrease the chance of injury.

CHAPTER 6

WORKOUT PLANS

12-Week Endomorph Workout Program

Weeks 1-3: Foundation Building

Day 1: Full-Body Strength Training

Squats: Begin with body weight or a light barbell. Focus on proper form and depth.

Push-Ups: Use a modified position (knees on the ground if needed) to build upper body strength.

Bent-Over Rows: Start with a manageable weight or resistance band.

Planks: Aim to increase your plank duration over time.

Day 2: Cardiovascular Exercise

Brisk Walking or Jogging: Start with a pace that challenges you but allows you to maintain proper form and breath control.

Day 3: Rest or Low-Intensity Activity

Day 4: Full-Body Strength Training

Deadlifts: Begin with light weights to master the technique.

Dumbbell Lunges: Use light dumbbells or just body weight.

Push-Ups: Aim for better form and control.

Russian Twists: Use a light medicine ball or dumbbell.

Day 5: Cardiovascular Exercise

Cycling or Swimming: Maintain a steady pace for 30 minutes.

Day 6: Rest or Low-Intensity Activity

Day 7: Rest

Additional Tips for Weeks 1-3:

Focus on proper form and technique to prevent injury.

Pay attention to your nutrition, ensuring you're eating a balanced diet and staying hydrated.

Gradually increase the intensity of your cardiovascular workouts as your fitness level improves.

Weeks 4-6: Progression and Intensity Increase

Days 1, 4: Full-Body Strength Training

Increase Resistance: Add 5-10% more weight to your strength training exercises.

Additional Set: Perform an extra set for each exercise.

Days 2, 5: Cardiovascular Exercise

Intensity/Duration Increase: Increase the intensity or duration of your cardio sessions by 5-10%.

Days 3, 6: Rest or Low-Intensity Activity

Day 7: Rest

Additional Tips for Weeks 4-6:

Continue focusing on proper form and gradually progress in your strength training.

Pay attention to recovery; if you experience excessive fatigue or soreness, consider more rest days or active recovery activities like gentle yoga or walking.

Weeks 7-9: Muscle Building and Definition

Days 1, 4: Full-Body Strength Training

Compound Exercises: Add compound movements like bench presses, pull-ups, and leg presses.

Core Focus: Incorporate core-strengthening exercises like planks, hanging leg raises, and Russian twists.

Days 2, 5: Cardiovascular Exercise

Intensity: Maintain high-intensity cardio workouts.

Interval Training: Consider structured interval workouts for an added challenge.

Days 3, 6: Flexibility and Mobility

Yoga or Pilates: Continue with flexibility-focused workouts.

Stretching: Focus on stretching major muscle groups to prevent tightness.

Day 7: Rest

Additional Tips for Weeks 7-9:

Emphasize proper nutrition to support muscle growth and recovery.

Stay consistent with your workouts and aim for progressive overload in strength training.

Stay hydrated and ensure you're getting enough protein in your diet to support muscle repair.

Weeks 10-12: Fine-Tuning and Fat Loss

Days 1, 4: Full-Body Strength Training

High-Intensity Strength Training: Focus on heavy weights and lower reps (6-10 reps).

Explosive Movements: Introduce explosive exercises like box jumps or kettlebell swings.

Days 2, 5: Cardiovascular Exercise

High-Intensity Intervals: Implement high-intensity interval training (HIIT) sessions for maximum calorie burn.

Days 3, 6: Flexibility and Mobility

Stretching and Foam Rolling: Continue to prioritize flexibility and recovery.

Day 7: Rest

Additional Tips for Weeks 10-12:

Pay close attention to your form, especially when lifting heavier weights.

Monitor your nutrition and consider a slight caloric deficit if weight loss is a goal.

Stay consistent, and if you encounter plateaus, consider varying your exercises or intensity to challenge your body.

Throughout the 12 weeks, remember the importance of rest, recovery, and listening to your body. Adequate sleep, stress management, and a balanced diet are crucial for your overall success. Additionally, stay patient and celebrate your progress along the way. After completing this program, consider transitioning to a maintenance plan to continue reaping the benefits of your hard work.

Evolution and Adaptation

In fitness and exercise science, progression and adaptability are important ideas. These ideas are essential for reaching and sustaining your fitness objectives, whether you want to develop strength, endurance, reduce weight, or improve your general health. Here's how progression and adaptation operate in the context of exercise:

Progression:

1. Gradual Overload: Progression is the process of gradually increasing the demands imposed on your body when exercising. This is sometimes referred to as "progressive overload." You stimulate your body to adapt and become stronger or more efficient by pushing it beyond its present limitations.
2. Increasing Intensity: You may progress by increasing the intensity of your workouts. This might include lifting larger weights, running faster or further, or raising resistance on cardio equipment.
3. Increased Reps or Sets: Increasing the number of repetitions (reps) or sets in your strength training routines is another approach to growth. For example, if you've been performing three sets of 10 reps for a specific exercise, you can increase to three sets of 12 reps or more.

4. Frequency: Increasing the frequency of your workouts can also help you grow. This entails working out more frequently each week or including extra sessions.
5. Change: Changing workouts, training regimens, or workout modalities might be considered advancement. For example, if you've been jogging, try cycling for a while to develop new muscle groups and avoid plateaus.

Adaptation:

1. Physiological Changes: When your body is consistently subjected to growing overload, it responds by undergoing physiological changes to meet the rising demands. Increased muscle strength, higher cardiovascular efficiency, increased endurance, and improved neuromuscular coordination are among the effects.
2. Better Performance: Adaptation leads to better performance. Exercises that were previously difficult will become easier, allowing you to lift bigger weights, run faster, or execute more reps with less effort.
3. Avoiding Plateaus: To avoid plateaus in your fitness journey, regular growth and adaptability are required.

Plateaus happen when your body grows acclimated to a certain amount of stress and stops progressing. You may prevent these plateaus by raising the intensity of your workouts or changing them up.

4. Injury Prevention: Proper progression and adaptation also aid in injury prevention. When your body gradually adapts to new demands, it has time to strengthen the muscles, ligaments, and joints, lowering the risk of overuse problems.
5. Long-Term Success: The keys to long-term fitness success are progression and adaptability. Whether your goals are short-term or long-term, these guidelines can help you stay on track and receive the advantages of regular exercise.

Periodization is an excellent method for implementing progression and adaptability. This is a systematic training technique that involves segmenting your training into several phases, each with a different emphasis on intensity, volume, and activity selection. Periodization aids in the prevention of overtraining, the reduction of the danger of burnout, and the optimization of outcomes.

Variation and cross-training

Cross-training and introducing variation into your workout regimen are critical techniques for reaching well-rounded health and fitness objectives. These methods can help you avoid plateaus, lower your risk of overuse injuries, and keep your training fresh and pleasant. Here are some ways that cross-training and diversity might help your fitness journey:

Cross-Training:

- Cross-training is engaging in a range of various sorts of exercise or physical activity rather than concentrating primarily on one. It enables you to focus on various muscle groups, energy systems, and movement patterns. Here are some of the advantages of cross-training:
- Overuse Injuries: Repeating the same motions or exercises daily can lead to overuse injuries. Cross-training lowers the risk of overuse injuries by resting particular muscle areas while activating others.
- Muscle Development: varying activities place varying demands on different muscle groups. Cross-training

promotes balanced muscle growth, which lowers the likelihood of muscular imbalances, which can lead to injuries or bad posture.
- Improving Overall Fitness: By participating in a variety of activities, you may enhance components of overall fitness such as cardiovascular endurance, muscular strength, flexibility, and agility.
- Cross-training gives a mental break from the monotony of the same program, which aids in keeping you intellectually engaged and motivated.
- Adaptation and Progression: When you change activities, your body must adjust to new difficulties. This adaptation can help you perform better in your major sport or exercise activity.

Variety:

- Variety within a certain form of exercise, such as strength training or aerobic sessions, can also be advantageous. Here are some ways that variation might improve your workout routine:
- Muscle Confusion: Changing your training program or workouts regularly keeps your muscles from adjusting too rapidly. This can result in increased muscular development and strength.

- Boredom may be avoided by repeating the same activities or regimens. Adding variation to training makes them interesting and pleasant.
- Different workouts are more helpful for achieving various fitness objectives. For example, complex workouts for strength and isolated exercises for muscle definition might be used.
- Exploring Interests: Variety helps you to try new things and find new interests in the world of fitness. You could discover that you appreciate hobbies you have never considered before.

Cross-training and a variety of examples:

- Cardiovascular training might include sports such as cycling, swimming, hiking, or rowing in addition to running.
- Vary your strength training regimen by varying the exercises, rep ranges, and equipment you employ. Bodyweight workouts, free weights, resistance bands, and machines should all be included.
- Flexibility and mobility can be improved by combining yoga, Pilates, and static stretching.

- High-Intensity Interval Training (HIIT): Switch between different HIIT routines, each with its own set of exercises and intervals.
- Participate in sports or leisure activities that you love, such as tennis, basketball, dance, or martial arts.
- Attend a range of group exercise courses such as spinning, barre, kickboxing, or dance aerobics.

CHAPTER 7

REST AND RECOVERY

Rest is Essential for Endomorphs

Rest is as vital for endomorphs as it is for people of all body types. A balanced and efficient fitness and weight control regimen includes enough rest and recuperation. Here's why relaxation is so important for endomorphs:

1. Muscle Regeneration:

Strength training is an important component of most fitness regimens, including those for endomorphs. Lifting weights or performing resistance workouts causes micro-tears in your muscle fibers. These tears require time to heal and regenerate, which occurs during rest times. Without adequate rest, your muscles will be unable to recuperate and expand, potentially leading to overtraining and injury.

2. Hormonal Harmony:

Rest helps to maintain hormonal balance, which is important for weight management and general health. When you sleep, your body creates growth hormone, which is important for muscular building, fat metabolism, and general healing. Inadequate sleep or rest might upset hormonal balance, thus impeding your weight loss attempts.

3. Overuse Injury Prevention:

Endomorphs, like everyone else, are prone to overuse injuries when they do not give their bodies time to recuperate. Overuse injuries can occur when muscles and joints are subjected to repetitive tension without proper rest. Rest days and varying training programs aid in the prevention of these ailments.

4. Energy Recovery:

Regular physical exercise can be physically hard, especially for endomorphs who are trying to lose weight. Rest days help your body to recover energy stores like glycogen, ensuring you have the stamina to keep up with your workouts.

5. Mental Rejuvenation:

Rest is important not only for physical healing but also for mental health. A well-balanced exercise regimen includes time for rest and mental replenishment. Overtraining can result in mental exhaustion, diminished motivation, and increased stress. Rest gives you a mental break and helps you stay motivated in your fitness path.

6. Support for the Immune System:

Exercising vigorously or for an extended time might temporarily deplete the immune system. Adequate rest allows your body to recuperate and promotes immune system function, lowering your risk of sickness and allowing you to stick to a consistent training schedule.

7. Long-Term Development:

Rest is an important part of long-term success. Consistency in your fitness path is more maintainable when regular rest days and recovery periods are included. This reduces fatigue and boosts your chances of meeting your weight loss and fitness objectives over time.

Rest and Recovery Suggestions:

Rest Days: Include regular rest days in your weekly training routine. These days can be spent completely resting or engaging in low-intensity activities such as walking or yoga.

Quality Sleep: Get 7-9 hours of quality sleep every night to help with muscle repair and general health.

On rest days, try engaging in light, non-strenuous exercises such as stretching, foam rolling, or leisurely cycling to improve blood flow and help in recuperation.

Pay attention to your food, especially post-workout nourishment. A proper diet aids healing by supplying vital nutrients to your muscles.

Pay Attention to Your Body: Overtraining symptoms include prolonged weariness, poor performance, and increased susceptibility to disease. As required, reduce the intensity of your workouts or take additional rest days.

Stay hydrated throughout the day, since dehydration can impede recovery and overall performance.

Strategies for Effective Recovery

Athletes, fitness enthusiasts, and people of all activity levels require effective recuperation procedures. Proper recuperation aids in the prevention of overuse injuries, improve performance and promotes general well-being. Here are some effective recovery strategies:

1. Sleep and rest:

Make sleep a priority, aiming for 7-9 hours of quality sleep every night. When we sleep, our bodies heal and renew tissues, regulate hormones, and consolidate learning and memory.

2. Active Rehabilitation:

On rest days, incorporate gentle, low-impact exercises. Walking, swimming, and mild yoga can all improve blood circulation, reduce muscular tightness, and help in recuperation.

3. Flexibility and stretching: Static stretches should be done after workouts to enhance flexibility and minimize muscular tension. Concentrate on key muscle groups, holding each stretch for 15-30 seconds.

4. Self-Massage and Foam Rolling: To target tight or aching muscles, use a foam roller or massage stick. This self-myofascial release method can help to relieve muscular knots and increase blood flow.

5. Hydration: Keep yourself hydrated throughout the day. Hydration is important for muscle function, nutrition transfer, and general recovery.

6. nutrition: Consume a well-balanced diet rich in protein to aid in muscle repair and development. Consume a post-workout breakfast or snack that contains both carbs and protein to restore glycogen levels and help recovery.

7. Heat and Ice Therapy: To relieve swelling and discomfort, apply ice to painful or inflamed regions (cryotherapy). Heat treatment (thermotherapy), such as applying a warm compress, can assist relax muscles and enhance blood flow.

8. Compression Wear: Compression sleeves or clothing can improve circulation, reduce muscular discomfort, and perhaps accelerate recovery time.

9. Nutritional Timing: To enhance muscle recovery, consume a balanced breakfast or snack including carbs and protein between 30 minutes to 2 hours of exercise.

10 contrasting baths or showers: Altering between hot and cold water in the shower or immersing limbs in hot and cold water baths might increase blood flow and relieve muscular pain.

11. Professional healing Modalities: For more focused healing and pain treatment, consider professional recovery methods such as massage therapy, acupuncture, or chiropractic care.

12. Mental Relaxation: To reduce stress and increase mental recuperation, use relaxation techniques such as meditation, deep breathing exercises, or mindfulness.

13. Avoid Overtraining: Listen to your body and avoid training loads that are too intense, which can lead to overtraining. Include rest days in your training plan.

14. Periodization: Use a periodization technique in your training to enhance recovery and adaptation by cycling through periods of varying intensities and volumes.

15. Gradual Overload: Increase the intensity and volume of your exercises gradually over time to allow your body to adapt and recuperate between sessions.

16. Monitor Progress: Keep a training notebook to keep track of your exercises, diet, and recuperation procedures. Adjust your strategy as necessary based on your progress and how your body reacts.

Stress and Sleep Management

Sleep and stress management are two essential components of general health and well-being. Both have a substantial influence on physical and mental health, as well as other elements of life such as fitness, productivity, and quality of life. Here's how to efficiently prioritize and manage sleep and stress:

Sleep Control:

1. Make Sleep a Priority: Make sleep a priority in your everyday schedule. To allow your body to relax, recoup, and regenerate, aim for 7-9 hours of excellent sleep every night.

2. Maintain a Regular Sleep Schedule: Every day, including on weekends, go to bed and wake up at the same hour. Consistency aids in the regulation of your body's internal clock.

3. Make Your Environment Sleep-Friendly: Make your bedroom sleep-friendly by keeping it dark, cool, and quiet. If necessary, consider utilizing blackout curtains and white noise machines.

4. Reduce Screen Time: Avoid using displays (phones, tablets, laptops, and televisions) at least an hour before going to bed. Screen blue light can interfere with your body's generation of melatonin, a hormone that governs sleep.

5. Relaxation Methods: Before going to bed, try some relaxation techniques like reading a book, moderate yoga, or meditating. These exercises might assist in relaxing your thoughts and preparing your body for sleep.

6. Maintain a Healthy Diet: Large meals, caffeine, and alcohol should be avoided close to bedtime. These can interfere with sleep habits.

7. Exercise regularly: Regular physical exercise might help you sleep better. Avoiding intense activity too close to bedtime, on the other hand, can have the opposite impact.

8. Restriction on Naps: If you must nap, keep them brief (20-30 minutes) and early in the day to prevent disrupting your nocturnal sleep.

9. Stress Management: Stress might interfere with sleep. To solve this issue, use stress management approaches.

Stress Reduction:

1. Determine Stressors: Recognize the stressors in your life. Work, relationships, money difficulties, and health challenges are all examples of this.

2. Time Administration: Set realistic objectives, prioritize work, and manage your time wisely. Time management alleviates feelings of overburden.

3. Meditation and mindfulness: To stay present and lessen anxiety, practice mindfulness and meditation. These approaches might assist you in dealing with stress in the present.

4. Physical Exercise: Regular exercise helps alleviate stress by generating endorphins, the body's natural mood enhancers.

5. Social Relationships: Maintain close social ties with friends and family. During difficult times, talking to loved ones and seeking assistance may be quite useful.

6. Relaxation Methods: To quiet your mind and lessen stress, try relaxation techniques such as deep breathing exercises, progressive muscle relaxation, or guided visualization.

7. Establish Boundaries: Set limits to safeguard your own time and space. When necessary, learn to say no.

8. Seek Professional Assistance: Consider obtaining help from a therapist, counselor, or mental health professional if stress becomes severe or chronic.

9. A Healthy Way of Life: To preserve general well-being, eat a balanced diet, exercise regularly, and emphasize self-care activities such as hobbies and relaxation.

10. Sleep: As previously said, emphasize excellent sleep hygiene because lack of sleep can worsen stress.

Maintaining physical and mental wellness requires balancing sleep and stress management. These techniques can help you perform better, stay psychologically robust, and live a better life. Experiment with different tactics to determine what works best for you, and keep in mind that seeking professional help for sleep or stress difficulties is always a good idea.

CHAPTER 9

ADDITIONAL CONSIDERATIONS

Endomorph Supplements

Endomorphs, like people of any body type, can benefit from supplements as part of a well-rounded diet and workout routine. However, it is critical to note that supplements should not be used in place of a well-balanced diet or a healthy lifestyle. They should support your overall health and fitness objectives. Endomorphs may benefit from the following supplements:

1. Supplements for protein: Endomorphs can benefit from protein supplements such as whey protein, casein protein, or plant-based protein to help them achieve their protein requirements, which are critical for muscle repair and development. Protein smoothies may be an easy post-workout snack.

2. BCAAs (Branched-Chain Amino Acids): BCAAs, which comprise leucine, isoleucine, and valine, can help in muscle repair and pain relief. They are frequently utilized by those who do strength training and strenuous activities.

3. Fatty Acids Omega-3: Omega-3 supplements, such as fish oil or algal oil (for vegetarians and vegans), can help reduce inflammation, promote heart health, and perhaps aid in weight reduction.

4. Vitamin D: Many people, including endomorphs, may be deficient in vitamin D. Vitamin D is necessary for bone health, immunological function, and general wellness. Consider having your vitamin D levels checked and supplementing as needed.

5. Calcium: Calcium is essential for bone health and may be especially advantageous for endomorphs, who are more likely to carry extra weight, putting stress on the bones.

6. Magnesium (Mg): Magnesium helps to maintain muscle and nerve function, bone health, and energy generation. It may aid in muscular relaxation and may lessen cramping.

7. Supplemental Fiber: While fiber is best obtained from whole meals, endomorphs who struggle with digestion or weight control may benefit from a fiber supplement.

8. Green Tea Extract: Green tea extract includes antioxidants and chemicals such as catechins, which may aid with fat reduction and metabolism. It is not a miracle cure, but it may be part of a comprehensive weight-loss strategy.

9. Pre-Exercise Supplements: Caffeine, beta-alanine, and nitric oxide precursors are common constituents in pre-workout supplements. They can deliver an energy boost and improve athletic performance. However, they should be taken with caution because some people are sensitive to stimulants.

10. Multivitamins: Taking a high-quality multivitamin can help address nutrient gaps in your diet, ensuring you obtain the vitamins and minerals you need for general health.

11. Probiotics: Probiotics can help with gut health, which is important for digestion, metabolism, and general health. A healthy stomach can help with weight loss.

Hormones and Weight Control

Hormones are important in weight management and general health. Understanding how hormones impact your body allows you to make more educated decisions about nutrition, exercise, and lifestyle. Here are several important hormones that affect weight management:

Insulin: Insulin is a pancreatic hormone that controls blood sugar levels. It aids in the absorption of glucose from the bloodstream for usage as energy or storage as fat. Insulin resistance, which occurs when cells do not respond effectively to insulin, can lead to weight gain and is linked to illnesses such as type 2 diabetes.

Leptin: Leptin is known as the "satiety hormone" since it tells your brain when you've had enough and should stop eating. Leptin resistance can occur in some circumstances, when the brain does not respond to leptin signals, potentially leading to overeating and weight gain.

Ghrelin: The "hunger hormone" ghrelin is generated by the stomach. It increases the appetite and alerts the brain that it is time to eat. Ghrelin levels that are too high might cause overeating and weight gain.

Cortisol: Cortisol, sometimes known as the "stress hormone," is produced in reaction to stress. Chronic stress can raise cortisol levels, which can contribute to weight growth, especially belly fat.

Thyroid hormones (T3 and T4): Thyroid hormones play an important role in metabolic regulation. Weight gain and difficulties decreasing weight can result from hypothyroidism, a condition in which the thyroid gland does not generate enough thyroid hormones.

Estrogen and progesterone are sex hormones that can impact weight management. Weight control in women can be influenced by hormonal shifts throughout the menstrual cycle, menopause, or hormonal diseases.

Testosterone: Testosterone is the predominant male sex hormone, but it is also found in lesser amounts in females. In both men and women, low testosterone levels can result in muscle loss, a slower metabolism, and weight gain.

development Hormone (GH): Growth hormone promotes muscular development as well as fat metabolism. Low GH levels, which are frequently connected with aging, might result in muscle loss and weight gain.

Adiponectin is a hormone generated by fat cells that aid in the regulation of metabolism and insulin sensitivity. Obesity and insulin resistance are linked to low adiponectin levels.

Catecholamines (Epinephrine and Norepinephrine): These hormones are generated during the stress reaction "fight or flight" and can temporarily enhance metabolism and energy consumption.

How to Manage Hormones for Weight Loss:

Balanced Diet: To assist hormone control, eat a well-balanced diet rich in a range of nutrients. Fiber-rich meals, lean proteins, and healthy fats can all help keep blood sugar levels stable.

Exercise regularly to enhance insulin sensitivity, increase metabolism, and reduce stress.

Stress Reduction: Use stress-reduction practices such as meditation, deep breathing, and mindfulness to keep cortisol levels under control.

Adequate Sleep: Make excellent sleep a priority, since lack of sleep can disturb hormone balance and increase hunger.

Hormone Replacement Treatment: In some circumstances, hormone replacement treatment under the supervision of a healthcare expert may be required to address hormonal imbalances.

Regular Health Checkups: Regular health checks can help discover and treat hormone imbalances or other health issues.

CONCLUSION

In summary, the "Endomorph Diet and Exercise Plan 2024" is a comprehensive guide tailored specifically for individuals with endomorphic body types. Throughout this book, we've explored the distinct challenges that endomorphs face in their fitness journeys and provided practical guidance to help them overcome these challenges and attain their health and wellness objectives.

Our journey began with an in-depth understanding of endomorph body types, highlighting the significance of acknowledging individual differences and the influence of genetics on our physique. Recognizing their unique body type empowers endomorphs to make informed decisions regarding their dietary and fitness strategies.

A recurring theme throughout the book has been the importance of personalized approaches. We've emphasized that there's no one-size-fits-all solution in the realm of health and fitness. Instead, endomorphs must tailor their approaches to align with their specific needs, preferences, and goals.

We've defined what characterizes endomorphs, including their propensity to store fat, rounded physique, and slower metabolism. This understanding serves as a foundational element in crafting effective diet and exercise regimens.

To lay the groundwork for a successful fitness journey, we've explored the process of defining health and fitness objectives. We've stressed the significance of setting clear, realistic, and measurable goals that encompass both short-term and long-term aspirations.

Setting realistic goals tailored to the endomorph body type has been a focal point. We've provided insights into establishing attainable targets for weight management, muscle development, and overall health enhancement. The emphasis has been on creating goals that motivate and can be sustained over time.

Monitoring progress and maintaining motivation have been essential aspects of our journey. We've discussed various methods for tracking fitness progress, from keeping journals to leveraging contemporary fitness technology. Staying motivated has been addressed through strategies such as seeking accountability, celebrating achievements, and adopting a growth-oriented mindset.

The core of the book lies in its extensive examination of nutrition and dietary planning for endomorphs. We've outlined endomorph-specific nutritional requirements, encompassing macronutrient ratios, calorie management, and the crucial role of nutrient-dense foods. The book offers a comprehensive guide to designing an endomorph diet plan, covering aspects such as meal planning, portion control, and fostering healthy eating habits that yield lasting results.

We've illustrated the practical application of these dietary principles through weekly meal planning, providing sample meal plans to assist endomorphs in making wholesome choices.

For those seeking a diverse range of recipes, we've curated a collection of breakfast, lunch, and dinner recipes complete with clear instructions and nutritional information. These recipes not only delight the palate but are also strategically crafted to support endomorphs in their pursuit of weight management and fitness objectives.

Navigating dining out and managing social occasions have been addressed with practical tips to empower endomorphs to make health-conscious decisions while savoring social interactions.

Transitioning to the exercise component, we've emphasized the pivotal role of physical activity in endomorph weight management. We've guided endomorphs in crafting an exercise regimen tailored to their needs, incorporating cardio, strength training, and flexibility exercises. A 12-week workout program has been provided as a structured blueprint for endomorphs to follow.

We've expanded on the fundamental concepts of progression, adaptation, cross-training, and variety to ensure that endomorphs consistently challenge their bodies while sidestepping plateaus and avoiding overuse injuries.

In closing, we've explored the significance of rest and recovery, along with strategies for effective recuperation. We've underscored that adequate rest is essential for muscle recovery, hormonal equilibrium, and overall well-being. Comprehensive recovery strategies have been outlined, spanning sleep management, stress mitigation, and self-care practices.

In essence, the "Endomorph Diet and Exercise Plan 2024" is an exhaustive manual that equips endomorphs with the knowledge, tools, and strategies required for a successful journey toward enhanced health and fitness. By embracing tailored approaches, setting practical goals, making informed dietary choices, and engaging in a balanced exercise regimen, endomorphs can realize their fitness ambitions and savor a healthier and more vibrant life. Remember, the key to success isn't just reaching your destination; it's about the journey itself, where each step taken represents progress towards improved health and well-being.

Made in the USA
Monee, IL
26 March 2024